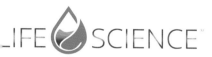

Copyright © 2018
Life Science Publishing and Hudson Leick
1.800.336.6308
www.DiscoverLSP.com

Printed in the United States of America
10 9 8 7 6 5 4 3 2 1

The essential and supplemental products discussed at length in this book are the sole product of Young Living Essential Oils, LC. The authors and publisher are completely separate entities from Young Living Essential Oils, LC. Products mentioned may be reformulated, discontinued, expanded, or enhanced by Young Living Essential Oils, LC at any given time.

Neither the authors nor the publisher advocate the use of any other essential oils without the Seed to Seal® guarantee. Even minor changes in the quality of an essential oil may render it, at best, useless and, at worst, dangerous. The use of essential oils should be done with thorough study, watchful care, and judicious prudence.

Much of the content in this book is derived from the Essential Oils Desk Reference, one of the most widely sought, sold, and read essential oils books of all time. This content is used with written permission from the publisher. Life Science Publishing retains all rights to the content of both the Essential Oils Desk Reference and all volumes in the Aroma series.

The material provided here is for educational purposes only and is not intended as diagnosis, treatment, or prescription for any disease, physical or emotional. The author, publisher, printer, and distributor(s) accept no responsibility for such use. Anyone suffering from any disease, illness, injury, or emotional distress should consult with a health care professional.

IN GRATITUDE

This book wouldn't have existed without the man Jeff Jensen, whose idea and trust in me brought it into reality. Kind thanks to the creative director Mark Richardson, for his patience and help. Most especially my thanks to my dear friend Mary Welsh whose love, support and time I most appreciate; with a keen eye for detail she has put thoughtful effort and her own generous nature into this very book. And lastly thanks to you dear reader, for being willing, open and curious to crack these pages.

In gratitude and Joy,

Hudson

TABLE OF CONTENTS

AUTHOR MESSAGE

Hi there!

My name is Hudson Leick, and I'm inviting you to take a journey with me into your world of emotions and the healing benefits of using essential oils. In order for you to get to know me better, I'm offering a sliver of my life and what has brought me to this particular place...

My life has been eclectic. My first job was modeling, starting at the age of 16, which took me all over the world. I then become a television and movie actress, garnering a small degree of fame. I write this not to brag, but in fact, to do just the opposite.

I learned at an early age that beauty, money, and fame did not bring me wholeness or even the Western World's idea of happiness, neither did it bring me the feeling of completeness. I was therefore forced (early-on) to find other paths to fulfillment. However, these jobs did teach me many things, and because they took me across the world, I was privileged to see and experience many diverse ways of life.

In this exploration, I began to study consistently many forms of yoga and meditation, and those have been my underlying focus for nearly 25 years. This passion enabled me to teach yoga classes and retreats for over two decades. I also found freeform dance, 5 Rhythms, and Soul Motion—and have been studying and teaching them for the last 18 years. But, my heart has been in my meditation practice, deeply for the last 11 years.

My search brought me to study for over 17 years with spiritual masters from across the world. Their inspiration helped me unlock my own capacity to offer spiritual counseling, which I do to this day. Most recently, I completed a yoga DVD and a meditation CD, that include the use of essential oils.

That said, I came from a very dark place in my teens and 20's, and I have worked very hard to bring light into myself and my world. This process of finding balance and enlightenment will never end for me.

I feel it is so important and beneficial to share what I have learned—not only for others who may be seeking light, but also for myself. That's because we are all in this together…this strange, wonderful, and precious life.

love sharing and teaching. I adore being around people who are willing and curious to learn and grow beyond the limits of their status quo. It takes courage to keep learning and growing, so I honor your willingness to pick up this book or any other book or modality for health and wholeness. It is a brave and self-loving act.

My intent for this book is for it to be a tool that leads to more self-acceptance, more balance, and in the end, more abundant love for yourself and others.

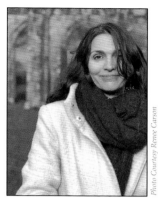

Photo Courtesy Renee Carson

When writing this book, I began by suggesting the oils that have so far, served me the best. To clarify: if you don't know where to start, please try my suggestions. But, as always regarding oils, this is a deeply personal experience. So please explore, in order that you begin to trust YOUR OWN intuitive healing process. Remember: in the end, only YOU know what feels best and works best, for your wholeness of self.

I want to take this time to welcome you to this book, and even more… hopefully, to a deeper connection to your most precious self!

With Warmth and Gratitude,

Hudson Leick

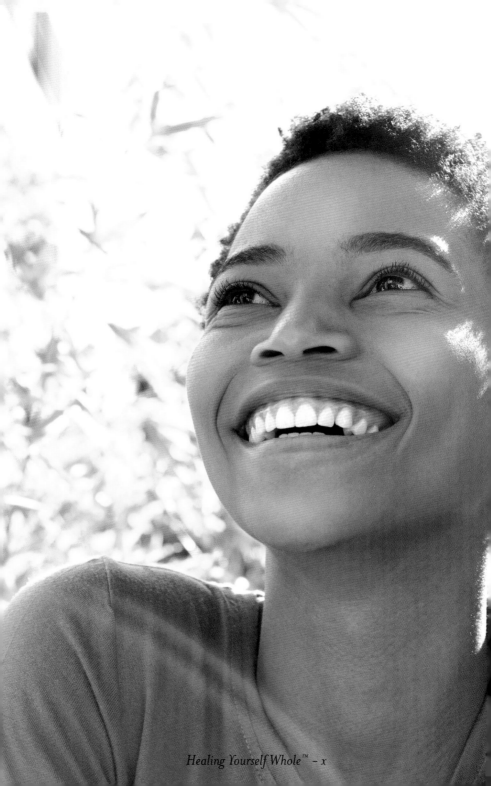

"The greatest glory in living lies not in never falling, but in rising every time we fall."

\- Nelson Mandela

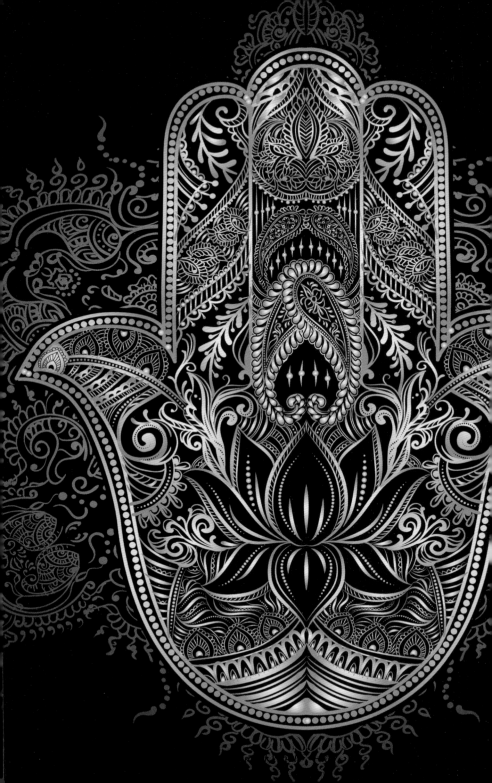

WELCOME

I would like to begin this book with a warm welcome! I appreciate your willingness and curiosity for your own self care and growth. Many sensitive people have been brought up with abuse, including neglect. I just want to take a moment to address this.

Whatever may have happened to you in the past was NOT your fault, but as a grown adult, it is now your responsibility to search for ways to heal. When I first heard someone say these words to me, I thought, "that is so unfair! Why do I have to do all the work?!" I feel differently about that now (most of the time). Now, I feel "I am so lucky I get to do this work and that I'm willing to do this work."

I have no ability to change any other human being but myself. We all can influence each other, yes, but only we, ourselves, can be willing.

I noticed how my unhealed, wounded self was affecting everything I came in contact with. So by doing the inside work first, I am able, with time to keep walking through life as a woman of grace more and more…

And, there will be no end to my growth as long as I can get up when I make mistakes, acknowledge them to myself and others, and keep on a path of willingness. I have come a very long way, and if I can do it, I know anyone can.

To walk this path of healing is not just a struggle or a life of having a cross to bear. I have had numerous joys and successes, new friendships and a deeper love for myself and others. I believe there are no accidents in life and the gift is by going through the pain. In fact, if these painful events didn't happen, I most likely would not be on this extraordinary path. In the end, I find the pains I've experienced not to be unfortunate. Furthermore, in time, I have found great gratitude for these exact experiences (as strange and as foreign as that may sound at first). They have caused me to find an indestructible light and a wellspring of love that lives with each one of us!

NOTE ABOUT PURITY

It is unfortunate that profit has taken priority over health. All too often, essential oils in the marketplace are diluted with solvents or chemicals. These synthetics and hybrids are not pure, nor are they natural. The essential oils we advocate in the Aroma series are only of the utmost, certified quality. We never advocate a product that may damage health or interfere with healing.

That said, essential oils have been used for thousands of years and have helped countless people to live healthier lives. As publishers of the most sought-after text about essential oils, the Essential Oil Desk Reference, we want to make as much information as easily accessible to you and the people you love.

It is with this spirit of education and sharing that we have compiled and summarized many of the specialized volumes in the Aroma series. Always take the time to read, study, and share the things you learn. Use good judgment as you add essential oils into your healthy lifestyle.

As Mary Young has said:

"Often times, we think we are helping someone by telling them what to do or giving them direction or advice about a problem that person may have. However, we take on a huge responsibility to give advice when we are not the expert or don't have the license that allows us to give advice. Besides that, if we give advice and then that advice doesn't work, that person may become angry with us and can accuse us of misdiagnosing, misunderstanding, and wasting their time and money.

In the world of essential oils, much information is available. If you are going to use any natural product, I suggest that you research all avenues possible and learn as much as you can for yourself, and then you be the one to decide how you will use any particular product.

It doesn't matter what you are going to eat, put on your skin, breathe, or even soak in, learning as much about your product is the most intelligent and safest thing you can do for yourself. The more information you have, the better choices you will make. After you study and research it for yourself, you may decide you don't want the very thing you thought you were excited about; but that is your decision, not someone else's decision about what you should do.

If you find something that interests you and you are uncertain, ask your doctor or someone educated in the field of health and nutrition. Ask their opinion to add to your knowledge bank. Look on the Internet to learn what research institutes, wellness centers, government agencies, the Surgeon General, and even the FDA have to say. You don't have to agree, but it is to your advantage to know what they say.

It is your responsibility to be responsible for yourself. It is your God-given right to search, read, study, and decide how you will feed and take care of your own body. Be independent and be wise."

--- From A Thought From Mary,
Mary Young 2016

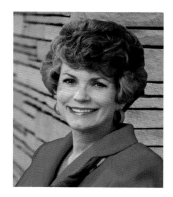

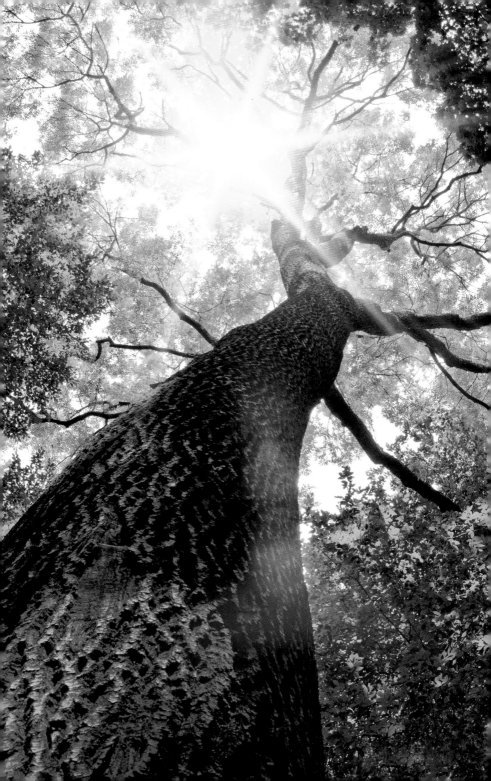

FEELINGS AND EMOTIONS

Some people might question whether or not we have a choice in how we feel. Large pharmaceutical corporations make a great deal of revenue from prescriptions that aim to help people manage their feelings. It is not my place to judge how a person chooses to handle their feelings. This book is about helping you discover your own individual path to balance.

My personal belief is that we have some choice in how we respond—and therefore, feel—while some parts of how we feel are individually ingrained. Overall, I believe we can make a choice to seek better ways of expressing our feelings and returning to a state of balance. We can always work to improve our lives. In this, it's best that we never stop.

However, I believe expressing emotions and making our feelings take a positive turn requires practice and has to be part of a larger plan for self-awareness.

I see each of us as having a unique fingerprint of experiences, thoughts, successes, failures, regrets, celebrations, and desires. We are complicated beings. There is nothing wrong with that. It's what makes each of us so beautiful.

In this book, we will use the terms "emotions" and "feelings" interchangeably.

"The best and most beautiful things in the world
cannot be seen or even touched. They must be felt with the heart."
---Helen Keller

Emotions are important. In many ways they are the spice of life. How can we feel hot without cold? How can we feel joy without knowing sorrow?

Emotions are a real expression of events and experience. We feel them as a response to something else. They are indicators that something is unbalanced or in the process of rebalancing. And, we cannot find balance by stuffing them in a box or putting them aside.

Our society tends to disregard emotions and can even label them a feminine quality and less desirable, or even unacceptable. One of the only "masculine" and acceptable emotions is anger and even that has limits.

The intent of this book is to allow for a brave and kind invitation to look and experience your own emotions, without labeling them good or bad. A useful analogy would be that they are just trapped energy units stored in our being. When we allow them to be expressed, we release them and work our way back to balance, which is a state of peace, calm, and serenity.

This process is one we will repeat throughout our lives. It's similar to an airline pilot. Due to variable wind and weather, the plane is actually consistently going off course from the ideal flight plan, but the pilot keeps adjusting—right, left, up, down—to stay on course.

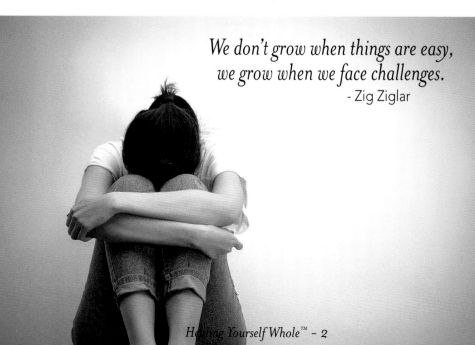

We don't grow when things are easy, we grow when we face challenges.
- Zig Ziglar

How to View Emotions

This is how I like to think of emotions. We will never be "rid" of them, we will never necessarily be at perfect peace as human beings, but if we get serious, we can find balance more and more quickly.

We, in this current culture, tend to be far from the connection of this earth and this is exactly the opposite of how our ancestors were. We no longer know how to grow crops, or know the phases of the moon, but we know how to get almost any information on our phones, at any time.

We are dominated by our mind and thoughts. We have a thought and we believe it to be "THE TRUTH." It may have truth in it, but more than likely, it's just downloaded information. It may or may not have any helpful wisdom for us.

Information may be interpreted in many different ways. It is up to us to create the filter, the interpretation, and the application for that information. This is where our feelings and emotions become important. When we find a balance between the head, our thoughts, and our intuitive feelings, we may better act from a more serene and simple place. We tend to experience this balance when we have a clear sense of what we are feeling. This helps us determine what our next action should be.

We stay super busy, so we don't have to feel. Some of us are so afraid to stay still, because if we do, we might start feeling a wave of emotions. That may be uncomfortable. We are afraid the feelings will never stop and maybe even destroy us.

Yet, if you think about it calmly, none of our feelings—or even all of them at once—can harm us. It's what we DO with our feelings or what we do to stop ourselves from feeling them that can cause us greater harm. In the extreme, we may cause self harm such as alcohol and drug abuse, cutting, or bulimia. Even excessive use of seemingly "positive" actions such as exercise, overworking, volunteering, and even spiritual practices can be something we do to distance ourselves from intimacy and true connection with our emotions.

Here's the good news...

This book can help. It has been designed for you to get to know yourself—to really learn to love yourself. Essential oils are a useful and inspiring tool to help you on your journey. I have suggested my favorite oils to enhance, stimulate, and magnify particular feelings. Alongside this, I offer specific instructions for placement on the parts of your body that best yield results.

These oil placements were discovered by experts in this field, and I am simply presenting what works for me. Remember, everyone is different and each human being—each life—is in constant growth/decay and change all the time.

So, there is no one thing to "cure what ails you." You can begin by asking yourself these questions:

- *What feelings do I struggle with in my life?*

- *What is the source of these feelings? Are they old? How old?*

- *Am I willing to have my feelings and have positive change in my life?*

- *Why do I feel I need to make a change?*

- *How will my life be more balanced, more joy-filled if I am willing to be open to positive change?*

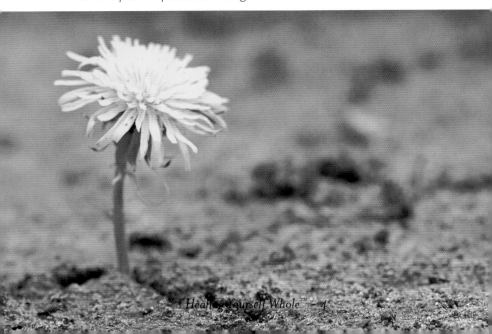

YOU ARE NOT BROKEN AND NEVER WERE...

There is an expression that I love. We are all alone in this, together. It is not meant to depress or scare you. It's just a profound truth. And, although we get a wonderful experience to love and engage with others, we do this work, this deep work alone. Even if we read this book as a group, we are doing it for ourselves. We are doing it alone—alone with spirit, nature, God, creation, the universe, whatever greater power you personally perceive.

During this process, you are only revealing, uncovering and re-balancing your own magnificence. I don't use that word lightly. I don't use it to feed your ego. We ALL are magnificent in myriad ways, yet all so different from each other. We only need to remember ourselves.

You are not any better or any worse than anyone else, and you are magnificent beyond your awareness. Let's see if we can re-awaken that realization and rediscover our very own self-love and sense of peace.

A great way to think of what's blocking us is comparing our vision to see to driving a car with a dirty windshield. It's smeared, and we can't see clearly out of it. However, the world is not dirty and neither are we. Rather, it is our perception that is temporarily marred. All that we need to do is to clean it. The blurred perception can also be called "stuck feelings," and they are the dirt that clouds our vision. Most importantly, if we are adamant about avoiding them over long periods of time, they can even make us very sick physically. So, just how do we clean them?

WHICH EMOTIONS?

We all suffer from fear, stress, and worry in our lives. But, in order to deal with them best, we need to understand our own willingness to make changes. This is a key word when evaluating your emotions: willingness.

It takes a willingness to be still with your emotions and allow them to come up. It requires a knowing that they will pass as you allow yourself to feel them, that there will be a natural endpoint. It also requires a knowledge that you do indeed have the ability to change your life.

Life just happens. A lot of us may have trauma from our past, including our upbringing. We drag this past, these early perceptions of the world, around with us. We perceive them through wounded, shattered glasses. It is not the truth, but it can become our truth. That's when it becomes a fixed way of relating to others and to the world around us. Most importantly, it becomes a fixed way of relating to ourselves.

Change...is an inside job

Acknowledging our pain, fear, vulnerabilities, our uncertainty of just what will happen next, will allow for more room in accepting the unknown. Seeing life this way, allows life to unfold.

When we are no longer reactive we can pause and take our time, allowing the possibility of a more fluid, heartfelt response. We experience a natural unfolding, rather than a heated reaction born out of habit and fear.

It also takes knowing that YOU are worth healing, and YOU really are the only one that can do it. However, this does not mean you have to do it alone.

There are many modalities of healing:
- Traditional (talk) therapy
- Physical activity, i.e.: yoga, swimming, dancing, walking, cycling
- Massage therapy
- Other modalities: cranial sacrum, chi gong, acupuncture, and acupressure

Whichever you choose, the main thing is that you yourself have acknowledged that you feel out of balance and that you are willing to try something different.

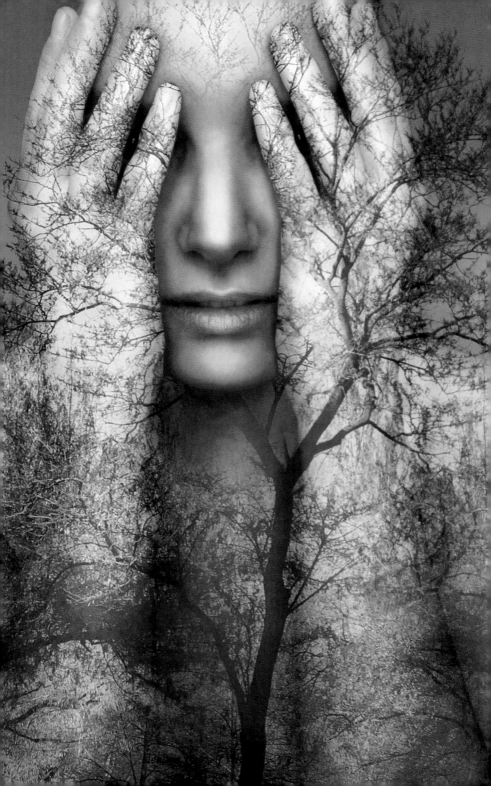

SELF-FORGIVENESS

You deserve your love and care. You are the only one that can give that to yourself. When you are willing to exercise self-forgiveness you grow the capacity to share it with others. And, it's important to note that only you can allow the love, care, and kindness that others offer to you as well.

Self-forgiveness is the ability to see your flaws openly and clearly and to let go of the ruthless judgment of self. Sometimes we are unable—or even unwilling—to see our own flaws. We might believe that we are made up entirely of these defects. Worse yet, we worry that if we admit them, the amount of guilt, shame, and remorse will be so overwhelming we will not be able to recover from it. Also, there can be the fear that if we expose our flaws to others, they will exploit us and use them as ammunition to attack and blame us—possibly over and over again.

Start with baby steps. Seeing our flaws, seeing just how harsh and demanding and judgmental we have been with ourselves is a great place to start. We are human, and we will never be a perfect being. Mistakes of all kinds can be forgiven—starting with our own.

We don't shout at or punish a baby for learning to walk when they consistently fall down. We can take this same gentle approach regarding ourselves. Yes, we have made blunders, mistakes, caused pain and hurt to others, and generally done so unknowingly to ourselves.

But here is the most important thing...you are worth forgiving. You deserve your love, tenderness, and forgiveness so that you can keep expanding and sharing your innate gifts with the world. And, you cannot do that while harboring resentment, dislike, and (possibly even) hate for yourself.

You are lovable, deserving, and worth your own freedom through self-forgiveness. No matter how many times you make mistakes, no matter what the mistakes, never give up. Keep trying. Keep kindly acknowledging your mistakes to yourself. Something that has greatly expanded my own self growth is to share these fallibilities with another person. Make sure that this other is someone who you respect, who is trustworthy and - most importantly - that you feel safe with. In time, if you stay open, you will change. It's inevitable.

FORGIVENESS OF OTHERS

Other humans can be challenging! There is an expression I adore, "be kind, for everyone you meet is fighting a hard battle." It's a quote from the turn of the century author Ian Maclaren (the pen name of the Rev. John Watson). It's a wise and loving quote, but hard in itself, when you feel someone has been unjust toward you or others.

Here's the thing. We have absolutely no control over other people. None. But, we do influence each other.

So, when you take care of yourself, when you learn how to love and accept yourself, you are actually giving permission for others to do the same. The only person you have any amount of control over is you. And, it always comes back to you. I don't mean this in an egotistical, narcissistic way. I mean this as you are responsible for you. The only control you have is over your actions, your words, your temperament. And, everyone else is also responsible for his or hers.

If someone else's behavior triggers emotions in you, it is important to know when to detach as kindly as you can. If we just stay in blame, we don't grow. Having said that, we don't have to be around other people that don't respect our boundaries or us. That is self-care. That is self-love.

Most importantly, keep in mind that everything and everyone changes. People have good and bad days. A person you may have difficulties with now could be one of your dearest friends later on down the road.

When we are really willing and able to begin this process, it will open up our world. We begin to see we have more in common with others than we have differences. Having said that, some people may be very challenging for you to forgive, but don't give up hope. This may take time. You may need to take very small steps. You might find you have to forgive yourself for not being able to forgive someone else.

If we force ourselves to forgive because it's the right thing to do, but our hearts don't yet feel it, then we will keep hating ourselves for failing. So, go gently.

Work first on yourself, allowing your human imperfection to be there and seeing if you can be willing to be willing to forgive. Also, forgiveness doesn't mean anyone can do or treat you any way they want. You may forgive someone, but take responsibility for yourself and don't place yourself in the same situation again with that person.

Discernment is important here, especially for people brought up with abuse

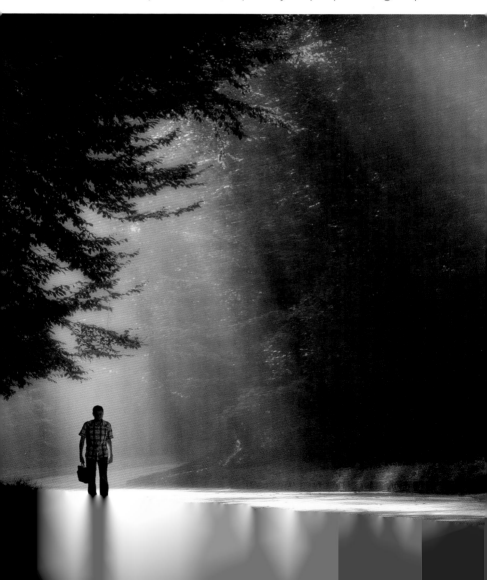

LETTING GO

Forgiveness is about being able to let go of anger you feel toward someone who has wronged you. It's about letting go of blame and realizing we all make mistakes. Someone else may have made a mistake. If wronging you was intentional, then what purpose does it serve to hold on to that anger?

Forgiveness is a conscious decision to release these feelings, to let go of resentment or vengeful thoughts toward the person who faulted you. When you make the deliberate choice to do this—and do it whether they deserve the forgiveness or not—you open yourself up to positive feelings. You make room in your heart to feel peace, balance, and even joy.

This process offers you peace of mind. You don't have to like the person. You don't have to love them or want to spend time with them or even come to a mutual closure. You simply have to let go of the pain, the hurt, the suffering, the anger, the hate, and the feelings of revenge.

Easier said than done, right? This will take some time. It takes effort. It takes a true and conscious choice on your part to let go of the habitual blaming thoughts.

When you are able to freely do this with ease (and this may take months, years, or even your whole life), you will find so much understanding and love of yourself. *That* is the gift of forgiveness.

It must all start with the willingness to forgive yourself. The shame/blame game all starts with being judgmental and cruel toward ourselves. We cannot jump to forgiving anyone else until we see how brutal we have been (and are) to ourselves.

BENEFITS OF USING AFFIRMATIONS WITH OILS

Affirmations help this entire process, giving it conscious and verbal expression of positive self-talk. They are a verbal expression of your innermost feelings. As you apply the oils, say the following phrases, preferably out loud (pick the ones that most resonate with you). Each time you do it, concentrate on your personal sincerity. If you don't feel sincere, say the affirmations with a desire to be sincere. Over time, this repetition will help you connect the thoughts to the feelings.

The goal is to reach a state of balance or release. Give it time and effort. It may take up to two weeks doing this 3 times a day to begin to feel this sense of release but have faith that it will come. Mark down any progress by tracking yourself. Remember it took time to form your current thoughts and emotional patterns. It will take time to change them. But know for certain IT IS POSSIBLE, and you and your life are so very worth it.

USING OILS

My favorite oil for addressing this issue is the Young Living blend, Forgiveness. Gary Young created this one to serve most people. If you don't have this blend, these singles can be helpful:

- Jasmine
- Rose
- Idaho Tansy
- Ocotea
- Jade Lemon
- Palo Santo

You can also use blends such as:

- RutaVaLa™ (regular oil or roll-on)
- Inner Harmony
- Harmony
- T.R. Care™
- Believe
- Common Sense™
- Humility™
- White Angelica
- Surrender™
- Joy™
- Oola® Faith™
- Divine Release™
- Release™
- AromaEase™
- Oola® Balance™

Placement

In addition to diffusion, directly inhaling from the bottle, or Vita-Flex points on the bottoms of the feet, I also recommend these placement points specifically for forgiveness:
- Navel
- Solar Plexus (the best way to describe this is where the rib cage comes together, just above the diaphragm)
- Heart

EXERCISE SELF-FORGIVENESS

Oil	Placement
Geranium	Place Geranium around the outside of the belly button and straight up the center of your body, to the solar plexus, then place more oil across the solar plexus.
Forgiveness	Place Forgiveness around the belly, on the insides of the wrists, and on your liver. Liver is the organ that holds anger and resentment.
Hawaiian Sandalwood	Place Hawaiian Sandalwood above and on eyebrows (careful around your eyes), and swipe across the middle of the forehead.

Repeat these affirmations out loud while placing your hands on the center of your chest (your heart center). Direct these words gently, lovingly and with conviction towards yourself.

Affirmations

As you apply your oils, say the following affirmations, preferably aloud - even better, in the mirror:

- *"I'm willing to let go of this pain, anger, and resentment."*

- *"It is safe for me to be free of this pain, anger, and resentment."*

- *"I free myself from negative emotional attachment."*

- *"I am so sorry. Please forgive me. Thank you. I love you."*

- *"I honor and love you."*

- *"I love you exactly the way you are."*

- *"I allow myself total and complete forgiveness for all past mistakes. I am worth loving."*

- *"My heart is free to forgive and be forgiven."*

- *"I forgive myself for being angry / impatient / un-thoughtful."*
  (Fill in the blank with your own habitual, negative way of behaving.)

- *"I forgive myself for not knowing better."*

- *"I allow myself to relax in a state of peace, and I release any harmful thoughts I have toward myself or others."*

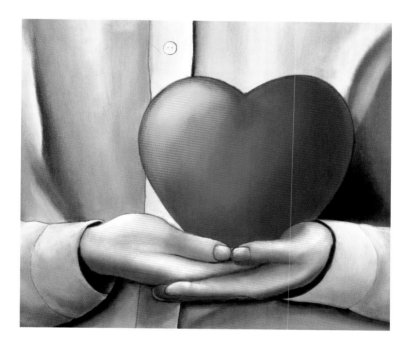

FORGIVING OTHER PEOPLE

As stated earlier, it is important to know when to detach as kindly as you can from something someone else may do that triggers you. If we just stay in blame, we don't grow. But, we do not have to be around other people that don't respect our boundaries or us. That is self-care. That is self-love. And, keep in mind, everything changes. Everyone changes. People have good and bad days. A person you may have difficulties with now, could be one of your dearest friends later on down the road.

Oil	Placement
Forgiveness	Place Forgiveness around the belly, on the insides of the wrists, and on your liver area.
Release	Place Release on your liver area.
Present Time	Place Present Time on your heart center and the insides of your wrists. (This is great for traffic. Use before heading into your commute.)
Clary Sage	Place Clary Sage on the soles of your feet and the palms of your hands.

Before you start, remind yourself that holding on to anger, resentment, and pain only (and always) harms us. Be clear about this fact before beginning your affirmations. Remember that you are doing this work to free yourself from all old, ugly, hardened emotions. It is your birthright to be free. You deserve to be free.

Affirmations

- "I thank all my pain, anger, and resentments, and I let them go."

- "It is safe for me to be free of all pain, anger, and resentments."

- "I surrender all negative emotional attachments I have towards others. They are free, and I am free."

- "My forgiveness heals me."

- "I forgive and release my childhood memories."

- "I let go of other people's mistakes as well as my own."

- "I send love and compassion out to the entire world."

- "I deserve total forgiveness."

- "I love and forgive humanity, including myself."

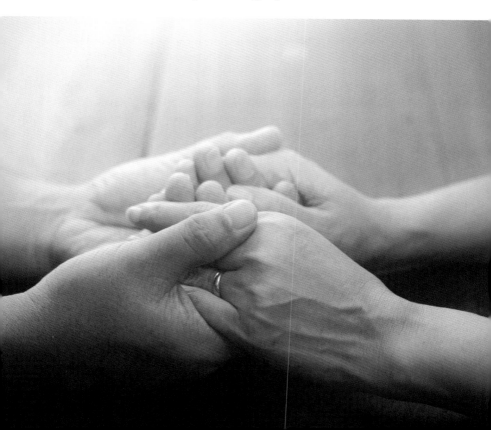

BE IN THE MOMENT

When I feel triggered by someone's behavior, it begins by my feeling quietl annoyed or angry. It can build, taking precious energy away from myself. If I am driving in a car, I might be so consumed with it that I even miss the freeway exit.

It is therefore extremely important to notice when you are upset or angry. Trying to get even is useless. Even if you do, not only is it exhausting, but it also feeds your own self-hatred. Such negative emotions in the end only harm you.

What I do:
I bring awareness to my mental thoughts and my overpowering feelings. When I am able to catch it, I stop myself and let go of it all and change my focus to simplicity, back to looking at my feet, the sky, or witnessing my breath.

Oils can also help with this process. Their scents can help your awareness as well as providing an opportunity to practice mindfulness.

When I am triggered with anger or impatience, I place Purification® above my breasts and below my collarbone. I then place Geranium on my solar plexus and Release all over my liver area.

This may be challenging, because other people may be around you. That doesn't matter. When you take care of your own energy, the energy around you may also change. I breathe into my solar plexus and cover it with my right hand, saying:

> *"I love you. You are okay. It's ALL okay, right here and right now."*

Say it as much as you need to, over and over. Hold your solar plexus with the tenderness of a parent holding an adored child. Stay with yourself as long as you need to. Feed yourself with this space and time. When you are alone, you can lie down on your back, placing your right hand over your heart and left hand over your belly button. Say (compassionately) "I love you, I love you, I love you," to really allow it in all aspects of your being.

RENDERING UNCONDITIONAL LOVE

Many of us never got the unconditional love we needed. By pausing and being in the moment, this allows us to give and receive it from ourselves. As before, using the oils helps with this process.

Oil	Placement
Rose	Heart
Frankincense	Belly Button / Hand in Hand
Gentle Baby™	Heart

Affirmations

- "I love you. You are completely loveable, and that love will never leave you."

- "Thank you for everything you provide for me, thank you...for you."

I prefer to do this as I'm going to bed, but it is fine to do it sitting up, if preferred. While I am lying on my belly, I have my left palm up and I lay my right palm over my left, facing down. My fingertips are at the center of each palm, my arms above my head with my elbows bent.

Focus your attention on the energy of both palms and fingertips in each hand, as you lovingly repeat deep gratitude for your being, for your precious life.

Our hands are how we hold, connect (shaking hands), comfort, give love, and create things for ourselves and others. When we focus on connecting this way, we share profound love and energy and the awareness of gratitude for ourselves.

Try using the oils before you go to sleep, repeating affirmations, and allowing yourself to deeply relax and receive your own appreciation and love.

EVERYDAY STRUGGLES

These are some of the most common emotions we all struggle with:
- Stress
- Worry
- Anxiety
- Fear

Stress

Stress is becoming more and more prevalent in modern life. The more our attention is pulled in different directions, with life demanding more and more from us, the more emotional strain we may feel. Our schedules become more hectic. We try to fit too much in a day to please everyone.

The exceptional thing about stress is that it can be caused by both good and bad experiences. As we cope with stress, it is important to identify the cause and be willing to consciously slow down. Nothing changes, if nothing changes. It's up to us to name it, claim it, and be willing to change it. While stress is hard on the mind and body, it really has a history in human behavior as well as our animal friends. It's part of a survival instinct, a biological response to potential danger. Our bodies are wonderful, complex vessels that often behave instinctively. Unfortunately, we tend to be overstressed in this modern-day culture. The fight or flight instincts were originally for our ancestors having to deal with life and death situations every day. Although we are now far from those times, our brains and body chemicals still react as though we are in extreme danger. This intense stress is magnified by caffeine and not at all useful in our everyday life.

Have you ever felt like your nerves were frayed? They most likely are. The good news is there are ways to learn how to relax—de-stress your mind, emotions, and body. Hopefully, this book will give you many different tools for how to do just that!

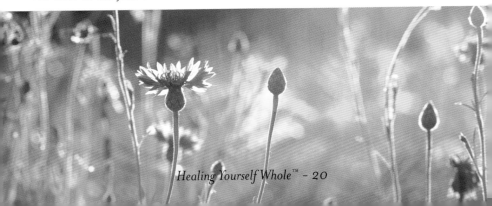

Worry

Much of our stress stems from worrying about things we can do nothing about, things we cannot control. We can become (both personally and as a culture) addicted to this kind of stress-tense, ultra-hurried, highly-caffeinated lifestyle.

Many of us suffer from the habitual "sickness" of believing "If I just keep thinking and worrying about this problem it will somehow help." Instead, we have to be willing to see our habitual ways of worrying and be open to stopping our "monkey mind." Just stop. Breathe. Release your shoulders, look up at the vastness of the sky, and remember you are not actually making the world turn. You have the right to relax an hour or even a minute. This practice will make a world of difference.

Anxiety

Anxiety is a close cousin to panic. We might feel fear of change—even if the change is beneficial to us—because it can feel stressful to do something unknown, something new. It can also manifest by just the feeling that life itself is moving too fast. Here are a few ways it shows up physically:

- Headaches
- Heart palpitations
- Sleeplessness
- Overeating
- Loss of appetite

In a more long-term way, stress and anxiety can affect us physically with stomach ulcers, shrinkage of lymphatic tissue and enlargement of the adrenals. Chronic stress can also lead to disease, such as heart attack, stroke, or cancer.

Fear

The feeling of fear can be crippling and debilitating. It is said that fear is at the root of most negative emotions. There are three primary opposites to fear: safety, acceptance, & peace. These opposites come into play depending on the source of our specific fear.

When the opposite of fear is safety (feeling secure), this means:
It is:
- Safe to be real
- Safe to feel the stress
- Safe to be imperfect
- Safe NOT to have all of the answers
- Safe not to have it all together
- Safe to admit failure, struggle, addiction, etc.

The opposite of fear is also acceptance. If we can accept whatever comes, if we can accept the present moment just as it is, if we can accept all our emotions about it, then we may be able to shift how the fear affects us.

Fear has another more positive side. It often helps us avoid danger, pain, or threats. To our ancestors (as it was noted before) this was critical in the hunting, gathering, farming, and physical world.

To us in the modern era, fear takes on a more consuming role. When it preoccupies our time and attention it draws away from our ability to achieve.

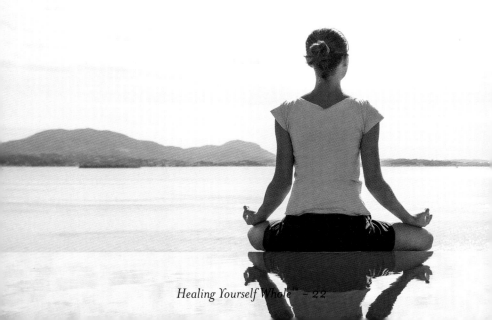

If we fear rejection, we may not speak up. If we fear failure, we may never try something new or step outside of our "comfort zone." Our life shrinks, so we can have more "control" over it. But, this fear can also take away our freedom to explore our lives, to shine, and to share our gifts with the world.

When the opposite of fear is peace, we can take a moment or two from out of our busy schedule and use it for personal reflection, exercise, meditation, stretching, and creative visualization. Take some time to try and still your mind. Focus on affirmations such as:

- *"I choose to feel internal peace and safety."*

- *"I choose to feel safe and protected."*

- *"There is always time for me."*

- *"I allow and embrace moments of deep serenity."*

- *"I am calm, relaxed, and peaceful."*

- *"In this moment, I don't need to be anywhere else, with anyone else, or doing anything else. I allow and absorb this moment of peace."*

In order to understand our emotions, we get the opportunity to embrace and accept them, without judging ourselves as being somehow "wrong" for having them.

ALLOWING

It is a good exercise to try welcoming our emotions, like we would a friend. Say to yourself "yes, I see you there." Simply breathe them in gently. As much as you can, accept them as a gift. Emotions are not an embarrassing weakness. They are not something you must get rid of as soon as possible. Vulnerability is not a sign of weakness, but instead, it takes great courage and strength to allow yourself to be still and to fully feel—even more if you are witnessed by another safe person.

Emotions will pass, as all things do. The more we can allow ourselves to acknowledge them and stay present with them, the more awareness we will have. In those moments, we are actually healing ourselves.

By continuing this practice, we may be able to help others through their difficult emotions. That's because we have done and continue to do our own work.

We can be present through simply doing nothing but witnessing without judgement. Yet again, using oils as part of our daily self-awareness practice will help focus our minds and hearts.

Remember:

- We don't need to fix ourselves.
- We are not broken.
- We inherit a lot of baggage from our family and our past.
- But, when we accept our emotions as they are, we have the opportunity to see ourselves and the world more clearly.

"Most humans are never fully present in the now, because unconsciously they believe that the next moment must be more important than this one.

SELF-RESPONSIBILITY

Even though we may reach the point where we accept and allow our feelings, it doesn't mean we have to let them control our actions. They don't have to negatively govern our lives.

This will take time and you may make a lot of mistakes on the way. When I say we don't have to react to them, I mean take out our negative emotions on others.

By doing this work, we get to let go of the shame and blame we put on ourselves when we have those feelings. We get to recognize, embrace, and fully feel them, but we don't have the right to spread our negative feelings across the world, directing those feelings at others. I say this not to have you go back to stuffing your emotions in a box and locking them away. I say this to encourage you to bring a higher self-awareness of your feelings into the light.

When we feel attacked and then attack back, the cycle never stops. The cycle continues. So, by you willing to do your part—your work—you then get to see when an interaction feels unhealthy, detach with love, and walk peacefully away from it. This not only helps you have better relationships, but it also helps spread kindness and awareness.

Speaking about taking responsibility...what has happened to you in life, in your upbringing, is not your fault. But now, as an adult, it is your responsibility (and only yours) to heal yourself. This empowers you to make positive changes.

But then you miss your whole life, which is never NOT now. And that's a revelation for some people to realize that your life is only ever now".
— Eckhart Tolle

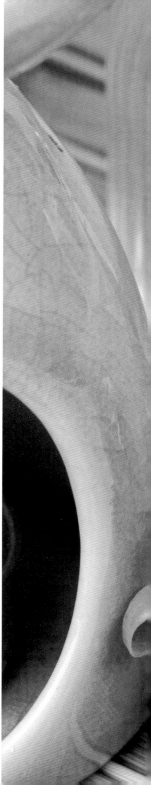

A HOLISTIC JOURNEY

As human beings, we are all greater than the sum of our parts. Likewise, we are all greater than the sum of our emotions. We are beautiful, complicated works of art.

By creating a balance towards our healing, we are accepting responsibility with a holistic approach towards our health, using preventive care and embracing as many modalities to help us in this process as we can. By living this holistic approach we become a more grounded, feeling and open human being, experiencing life in a more efficient, balanced and calm way.

"Everything changes when you start to emit your own frequency rather than absorbing the frequencies around you, when you start imprinting your intent on the universe rather than receiving an imprint from existence."
— Barbara Marciniak

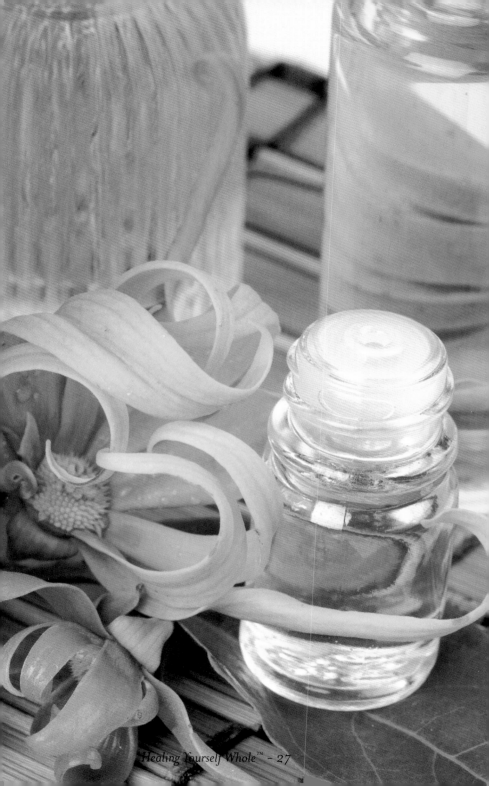

DISCOVERING YOU

Answer these questions and write the answers quickly without overthinking. If these pages are too small and limit your free form writing, buy a notebook especially for this work.

Set a timer for 15-30 minutes. Try to write free-flowing without over-thinking and without taking the pen off the paper. After you finish with all questions and your answers, my suggestion is to find a trusted person to read your answers out loud to, someone you feel safe with. It can be a spouse, friend, therapist, or trusted spiritual leader. Read them aloud to another so that you may be witnessed—and also hear for yourself. This is incredibly healing. It may not feel as helpful if you're just writing it alone. When you take the opportunity to read it to another, something changes. That witnessing can help us feel ourselves more clearly.

You've come this far. You have nothing to lose but your habitual ways of feeling bad and stuck! Give it a go! I'm cheering you on from here!

Be as honest as you can in answering these questions:

- Which emotions do you most struggle with?
- Do you have a lot of anger, resentment or even hatred?
- Are you overly worried, anxious or stressed out?
- Are you consistently depressed?
- Are you low on energy?

_____

_____

_____

_____

_____

_____

_____

_____

_____

_____

- Do these emotions keep you from achieving your best every day?
- Do they prevent you from having a meaningful relationship?
- Do they interfere with your ability to feel appreciation for life?
- Describe how they make you feel.

_____

_____

_____

_____

_____

_____

_____

_____

_____

_____

_____

_____

_____

_____

_____

_____

_____

_____

_____

_____

- What do you most appreciate about your life?
- What do you most appreciate about your body, your mind, your health?
- What do you most appreciate in the ones you love?
  (suggestion: be willing to share this information with them)

PERSONAL INVENTORY

Make a list of the emotions you would like to acknowledge, express and accept. Maybe they manifest or bubble to the surface in inappropriate ways. Or, maybe you feel locked-down, as if you don't have the right to feel them. Regardless of how you currently experience them, make a list of what they are, how they manifest, and your own healthy active solutions to help heal. Here's an example:

Emotion	*How it manifests…*	*How can I acknowledge this feeling fully in a healthy way?*
Anger	I hold onto resentment towards a person and ignore them to punish them	Write about the specific interaction and see my anger, ask why was I angry, be willing to have a conversation with the other person. Owning my anger about the situation and apologizing for my reaction of icing the other person out and wanting to punish them.

_____

_____

_____

_____

_____

_____

_____

_____

_____

_____

_____

_____

_____

_____

_____

_____

_____

EMOTIONAL SUPPORT WITH ESSENTIAL OILS

The Essential Oils Desk Reference is a great resource for exploring emotions with essential oils. I recommend buying one if you are serious about using essential oils to help re-balance your emotional life. It's an incredibly helpful and clear book.

I've adapted this section from the Desk Reference for you to have a quick guide when you need to explore your oils with your emotions. These oils are exclusively from Young Living Essential Oils, which are the oils I use, work with and believe in. But please don't let that stop you. Use other oils if you have them, but make sure they are pure and well-made. I will add, though, I have not yet found another essential oil to be better than Young Living. To me, this brand is the finest. They have the unique profile that fully helps support you in creating a personal emotional healing pathway.

Here is a small list of the oils I suggest. If you are new to oils you can try these to start, but please remember, everyone is different. Eventually, branch out and trust your own innate intuition.

Abuse

Singles: Geranium, Ylang Ylang, Palo Santo, Ocotea, Frankincense, Sacred Frankincense

Blends: SARA™, Hope™, Freedom™, Joy, Peace & Calming®, Inner Child, AromaSleep™, SleepyIze™, Grounding™, Trauma Life, Divine Release, Release, Valor, Valor® Roll-On, Valor II, Forgiveness, White Angelica

Agitation

Singles: Jade Lemon, Clary Sage, Frankincense, Sacred Frankincense, Geranium, Rose, Ylang Ylang

Blends: Peace & Calming, Peace & Calming™ II, Valor, Valor Roll-On, Valor II, Tranquil Roll-On, Harmony, Forgiveness, Australian Blue™

Anger

Singles: Idaho Blue Spruce, Cedarwood, Sacred Frankincense, Lavender, Myrrh, Orange, Rose, Roman Chamomile, Ylang Ylang

Blends: Release, Valor, Valor Roll-On, Valor II, Sacred Mountain™, Harmony, Hope, Forgiveness, Transformation, Present Time, Tranquil Roll-On, Surrender, Christmas Spirit™, White Angelica

Anxiety

Singles: Idaho Blue Spruce, Orange, Roman Chamomile, Lavender, Sacred Frankincense, Frankincense, Clary Sage, Jade Lemon

Blends: Freedom, Valor, Valor Roll-On, Valor II, Hope, Peace & Calming, Tranquil Roll-On, Joy, Present Time, Abundance™, Surrender, Shutran, White Angelica, Australian Blue

Apathy

Singles: Frankincense, Sacred Frankincense, Geranium, Jasmine, Orange, Peppermint, Rose, Sandalwood, Jade Lemon, Thyme, Lime

Blends: Joy, Harmony, Valor, Valor Roll-On, Valor II, 3 Wise Men™, Hope, Believe, Motivation™, Live with Passion, Highest Potential™, Shutran

Argumentative

Singles: Idaho Blue Spruce, Cedarwood, Palo Santo, Sacred Frankincense, Jade Lemon, Jasmine, Orange, Ylang Ylang

Blends: Peace & Calming, Peace & Calming II, Egyptian Gold, Harmony, Valor, Valor Roll-On, Humility, Release

Boredom

Singles: Cedarwood, Black Pepper, Roman Chamomile, Sacred Frankincense, Juniper, Lavender, Rosemary, Jade Lemon, Thyme

Blends: Dream Catcher™, Citrus Fresh, Motivation, Transformation™, Valor Roll-On

Concentration

Singles: Cedarwood, Juniper, Lavender, Lemon, Basil, Helichrysum, Orange, Peppermint, Sandalwood

Blends: Clarity™, Highest Potential, Gatheringý, Dream Catcher, Citrus Fresh, Magnify Your Purpose™

Confusion

Singles: Cedarwood, Peppermint, Sacred Frankincense, Ginger, Rosemary, Basil, Thyme, Ylang Ylang

Blends: Clarity, Citrus Fresh, Common Sense, Harmony, Valor, Valor Roll-On, Valor II, Abundance

Depression

Singles: Sacred Frankincense, Idaho Blue Spruce, Palo Santo, Jade Lemon, Lemon, Sandalwood, Geranium, Lavender, Grapefruit, Lime, Pine

Blends: Valor, Valor Roll-On, Valor II, Motivation, Live with Passion™, Believe, Christmas Spirit, Shutran, Citrus Fresh, Sacred Mountain, Joy, Australian Blue, Dragon Time™, Gentle Baby, SARA

Despair

Singles: Cedarwood, Northern Lights Black Spruce, Sacred Frankincense, Idaho Blue Spruce, Lavender, Geranium, Jade Lemon, Lemon, Orange, Peppermint, Rosemary

Blends Joy, Believe, Christmas Spirit, Harmony, Gathering, Grounding, Inner Child, Forgiveness, Abundance, Australian Blue, Gentle Baby, SARA

Disappointment

Singles: Sacred Frankincense, Palo Santo, Geranium, Ginger, Juniper, Tangerine

Blends: Hope, Joy, Christmas Spirit, Valor, Valor Roll-On, Valor II, Dream Catcher, Divine Release, Magnify Your Purpose, Australian Blue, Gentle Baby

Discouragement

Singles: Idaho Blue Spruce, Bergamot, Cedarwood, Geranium, Dalmatia Juniper, Lavender, Cardamom, Nutmeg

Blends: Valor, Valor Roll-On, Valor II, Shutran, Sacred Mountain, Dream Catcher, Citrus Fresh, En-R-Gee

Fear

Singles: Palo Santo, Roman Chamomile, Geranium, Juniper, Northern Lights, Black Spruce, Jade Lemon, Cistus

Blends: Valor, Valor Roll-On, Valor II, The Gift, Tranquil Roll-On, Australian Blue, Christmas Spirit

Forgetfulness

Singles: Cedarwood, Roman Chamomile, Sacred Frankincense, Rosemary, Peppermint, Thyme

Blends: Clarity, Valor, Valor Roll- On, Valor II, Present Time, 3 Wise Men, Egyptian Gold

Frustration

Singles: Ginger, Lavender, Orange, Peppermint

Blends: Valor, Valor Roll-On, Valor II, Sacred Mountain, 3 Wise Men, Humility, Peace & Calming, Peace & Calming II, Australian Blue

Grief/Sorrow

Singles: Bergamot, Palo Santo, Roman Chamomile, Clary Sage, Eucalyptus Globulus, Melissa

Blends: Valor, Valor Roll-On, Valor II, Inner Child, Harmony, Present Time, Australian Blue, SARA

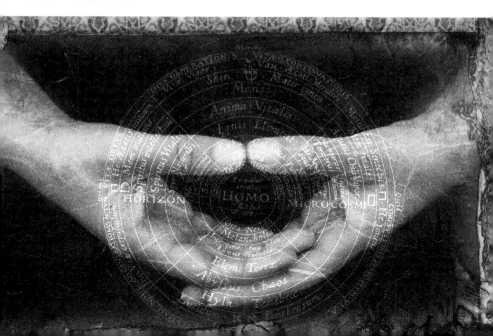

Guilt

Singles: Roman Chamomile, Geranium, Sacred Frankincense, Rose, Thyme

Blends: Valor, Valor Roll-On, Valor II, Inspiration™, Harmony, Present Time, Egyptian Gold, SARA

Irritability

Singles: Roman Chamomile, Palo Santo, Jade Lemon, Tangerine,

Blends: Valor, Valor Roll-On, Valor II, Peace & Calming, Peace & Calming II, Release, Surrender, Transformation, Dragon Time, Lady Sclareol™

Jealousy

Singles: Palo Santo, Dorado Azul™, Sacred Frankincense, Orange, Rose

Blends: The Gift™, Sacred Mountain, Humility, Surrender, Release, Gratitude™

Mood Swings

Singles: Idaho Blue Spruce, Clary Sage, Sage, Geranium, Fennel, Lavender, Peppermint, Rose, Jasmine

Blends: Peace & Calming, Peace & Calming II, Valor, Valor Roll-On, Valor II, Dragon Time, Mister™, White Angelica, Australian Blue, Shutran, Lady Sclareol

Obsessiveness

Singles: Clary Sage, Palo Santo, Geranium, Lavender, Ylang Ylang, Patchouli

Blends: Sacred Mountain, The Gift, Acceptance, Inner Child, Surrender, Release

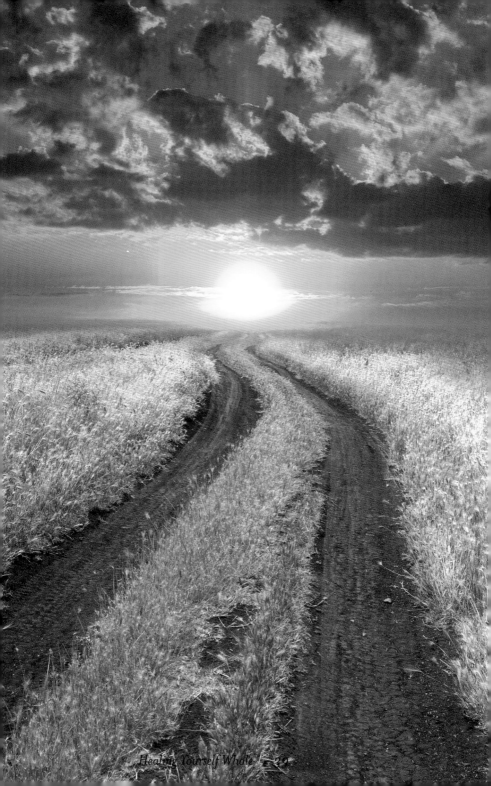

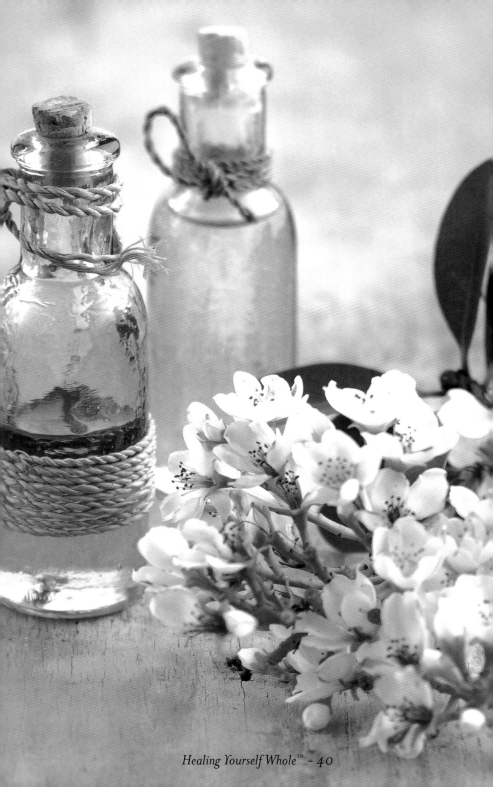

Panic

Singles: Fennel, Roman Chamomile, Myrrh, Sacred Frankincense, Lavender,

Blends: Valor, Valor Roll-On, Valor II, Peace & Calming, Peace & Calming II, Grounding, Shutran, Australian Blue

Resentment

Singles: Jasmine, Rose, Idaho Tansy, Palo Santo

Blends: Forgiveness, Harmony, Humility, White Angelica, Surrender, Release

Shock

Singles: Helichrysum, Basil, Roman Chamomile, Rosemary, Cardamom

Blends: Clarity, Chivalry, Inspiration, Tranquil Roll-On, Grounding, Australian Blue

Stress

Singles: Idaho Blue Spruce, Roman Chamomile, Sacred Frankincense, Cardamom, Cedarwood, Melissa, Lime, Clove

Blends: Tranquil Roll-On, Christmas Spirit, Citrus Fresh, Highest Potential, Transformation, White Angelica

Adapted from the Essential Oils Desk Reference, 7th Edition. Used with permission.

THE FEELINGS™ COLLECTION
from Young Living

It would be incomplete of me to write about emotions and feelings without highlighting the Feelings collection from Young Living. This kit contains six essential oil blends that Gary Young formulated to help us manage our emotional wellbeing. They are primarily for diffusion, but I find they can be a great support when applied topically. Please note, always use oils topically by blending them with a carrier oil eg sweet almond oil, coconut oil, jojoba oil etc.

The kit has its own set of instructions, but I have also explored and chronicled my own experiences using these oils.

They can be used throughout the day to help support you in your efforts to integrate and balance your emotions.

As you seek to explore your emotions, you may find that some oils work better for you than others, depending upon the time in your life, where you are in your journey for healing, and how much you've experienced and recognized about yourself.

There are many oils that are nice to have on hand as you explore this part of your life. I particularly recommend the Feelings collection from Young Living to help support and enrich you on your journey to more self-awareness.

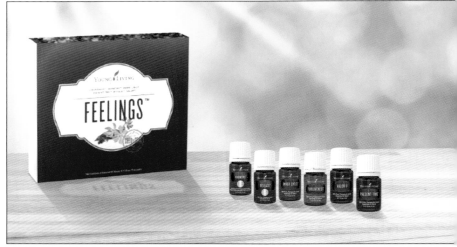

The Feelings Collection Includes:

- Harmony™, 5 ml

This is one of the most powerful, spiritual and emotional blends, comprising 17 therapeutic-grade oils. Each of these oils works on its own to help us with emotional support; however, the blend together is greater than the sum of its parts. Harmony helps bring balance to the energy centers of our body. It's also good for freeing up emotional blocks to allow natural energy to flow freely through our bodies. It is uplifting and elevating to the mind, helping to support a positive attitude.

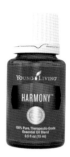

- Forgiveness™, 5 ml

Fifteen essential oils work in tandem to provide you with calming, balancing, relaxing, cleansing, soothing, and purifying emotional support. It is especially good for releasing such negative emotions as betrayal, revenge, and distrust. It helps you to open up alternative emotional pathways so that it becomes easier to move past negative patterns, forgive wrongs or hurts, and release the negative memories associated with them.

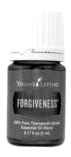

- Inner Child™, 5 ml

Through the course of our lives, many of us forget our inner child or inner self. When we suffer emotional abuses or mistreatment, we often cover our core with an artificial sense of self fueled by blame and resentment. This unique blend supports you in accepting your present life, letting go of the blame, and re-connecting with your inner core. It helps to release emotional patterns and develop a new, fresh outlook on life. It's perfect for helping you embrace a new perspective as you delve deeply into who you really are. It has a calming, nurturing, comforting fragrance—one that helps you care for yourself in a gentle way.

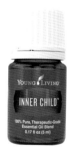

- Present Time™, 5 ml

This marvelous blend is about being truly in the moment. Many of us experience anxiety about the past or future—so much so, that we fixate on those moments rather than the one we're in. When we live in the moment, we can actually bring about emotional change. When we dwell on the past or fixate on the future, we turn to things outside of our control. We desperately cling to a sense of other, a series of emotions that may paralyze us. Being present allows us the necessary grounding it takes to look at what we would like to change and take action to change it.

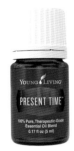

- Release™, 5ml

The 16 oils in this blend unite to help you let go of anger and frustration. This helps release deep-seated trauma and anger in order to heal and support emotional wellbeing. Many people find that oils which help with cleansing (SARA and Inner Child) and clarity (Brain Power™, Clarity, Peppermint) are effective when used in conjunction with Release. That's because just opening the anger and negative emotions may not be enough to clear the mind and body of the detrimental effects.

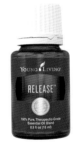

- Valor II™, 5 ml

This rare and remarkable blend contains 11 exclusive Young Living essential oils that connect us with our inner inspiration, calmness, strength, and courage. The empowering constituents help balance energies and instill courage, confidence, and self-esteem.

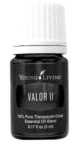

GETTING STARTED WITH THE FEELINGS KIT

This kit was the first experience I had with Young Living oils. I used several of the oils in this collection immediately.

In addition to the oils, the kit comes with a very informative CD that suggests not only where to use the oils, but also details how the Ancient Egyptians used them. There's also a good deal of information describing how Young Living built the current distilling process on that ancient tradition.

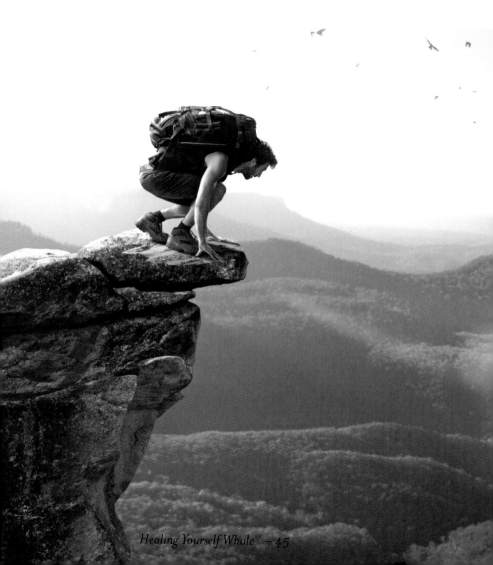

FEELINGS KIT BLEND: HARMONY

"Happiness is when what you think, what you say,
and what you do are in harmony."
– Gandhi

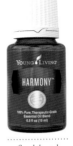

I adore this aroma! It is very grounded yet incredibly light at the same time. I use this oil not only for when I need to interact with others, but I also use it first for a better relationship with myself.

Sandalwood
Lavender
Ylang Ylang
Frankincense
Orange
Angelica
Geranium
Hyssop
Spanish Sage
Spruce
Coriander
Bergamot
Lemon
Jasmine
Roman Chamomile
Palmarosa
Rose

Harmony Placements

I use Harmony on my heart center, the insides of my ankles, a swipe across the back of my neck, and behind my earlobes (following from the top to the bottom behind ears).

I find the energies in this oil to be hopeful and it gives me a sparkling "clean" feeling when I use it.

I will also either swipe a bit under my nose (not for everyone as this oil may be too strong for extremely sensitive skin) or I hold it in front of my nose for 1-2 minutes breathing slowly and deeply, relaxing my shoulders and taking in the word Harmony. In these deliberate moments, I focus on allowing myself to integrate all aspects of myself, accepting myself to be a precious and divine soul—not important or unimportant—just a small valuable piece of the whole of creation.

Harmony Affirmations

- *"I am willing to live life with ease."*

- *"I will not be afraid to show kindness and love."*

- *"I am kind and loving."*

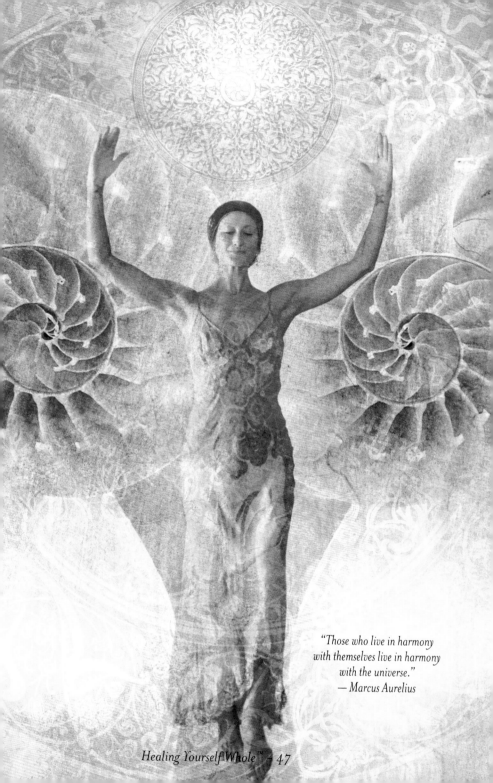

"Those who live in harmony
with themselves live in harmony
with the universe."
— Marcus Aurelius

FEELINGS KIT BLEND: FORGIVENESS

"Forgiveness is a virtue of the brave."
— Indira Gandhi

Forgiveness smells earthy, a little musky, and very grounding to me. This strong blend of oils creates a base for one to feel more stable. It is incredibly important to feel that strong grounding so that you can focus on the deep work of self care. I believe the first person we must always forgive is ourself, because it is from (at times) that place of our own distorted self-perception that we tend to act out on the rest of the world.

So, use this oil to release yourself from shame, self-hatred, perfectionism, self-judgement and whatever else blocks you from feeling whole. This oil supports you in going from those emotions to feeling loved and lovable.

We all do the best we can in each moment. But, with more awareness, more forgiveness, we have more space to make better choices with how we treat ourselves and how we treat others.

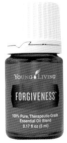

Melissa
Geranium
Frankincense
Sandalwood
Coriander
Angelica
Lavender
Bergamot
Lemon
Ylang Ylang
Jasmine
Helichrysum
Roman Chamomile
Palmarosa
Rose

Forgiveness Placements

I apply Forgiveness to the navel to start with, a way to approach forgiveness daily. If I am struggling with forgiving someone or with a particular issue, I go a little deeper. I will often begin by smelling the bottle for 1-2 minutes.

Other places to apply the oil are on the shoulders, back of the ears, throat, spine, wrists, neck and/or feet.

Please keep in mind that by your willingness to let go of your own pains and judgements you open yourself up to experience new and great things in life.

Forgiveness Affirmations

- "The past is complete. I live in the present."

- "I choose to live in the now and create my future. The past has no bearing on my present."

- "I allow others to live their lives as I will live mine."

- "I allow myself to make mistakes and learn from them."

- "I allow others to make mistakes."

- "I forgive myself for holding a grudge."

- "I forgive my parents and my family for any wrongs they've done me—either knowingly or unknowingly."

- "As I forgive myself, I find greater abundance for forgiving others."

- "I see each day as an opportunity and I begin it with a fresh, clean slate."

- "I move beyond forgiveness to understanding, and I have kindness and compassion for all."

- "I am forgiving, loving, gentle, kind, and safe, and I know that the universe loves me."

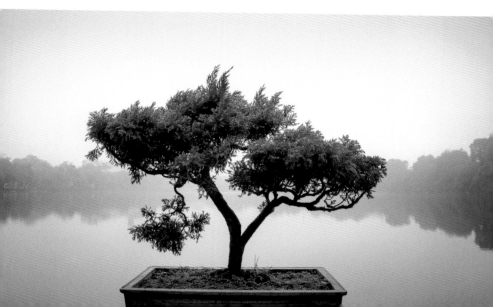

FEELINGS KIT BLEND: INNER CHILD

*"Sometimes what you're most afraid of doing is the
very thing that will set you free."*
- Robert Tew

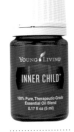

Orange
Tangerine
Ylang Ylang
Jasmine
Sandalwood
Lemongrass
Spruce
Neroli

A lot of us were neglected or abused as children. Even if we didn't suffer active neglect or abuse, we may not have been as nurtured as we could have been. We may not have had a sufficient experience with what true nurturing and support felt like. If we lack this important emotional component, we may not be able to nurture ourselves or others.

As adults we can continue to treat and talk to ourselves the same way as we were spoken to as children. It may be so habitual you don't even see it. But, when we slow down with ourselves enough, it is possible to get a glimpse of how hard—or even cruelly—we treat ourselves.

Inner Child was one of the first mixed oils I ever tried. I was immediately drawn to the aroma, which is fresh, warm, light and somehow very comforting. Our inner child is the source of our vitality and creativity. It is our pure sense of wonder to be able to create from nothing. Start slowly and gently, as you would with any child. Use the oils and affirmations as much as you feel you need to during your day. Don't be afraid to really put the focus on yourself in a gentle loving way. It took time to develop your negative thoughts and it will take some time to heal them.

Know that you CAN heal.
You are WORTH healing.
You are LOVABLE!

Inner Child Placements

Place it on the temples, rims of ears, wrists and on thumb, to suck. (Now, this may seem wild and crazy, but I do, in fact, do this myself.) Wash your hands, apply 1 to 2 drops on your right thumb and put the whole thumb in your mouth and suck on it for 1 to 3 minutes, depending on your mood. (Note: I do not however, do this in public! Although...to each his own.) Not surprisingly, thumb sucking is very calming and nurturing.

When I first heard other emotional essential oil experts speak about this practice I was dubious at first. However, I thought nothing ventured, nothing gained. So, being willing to try it myself, I now see how helpful it can be, not to mention it also tastes great.

Inner Child Affirmations

Our inner child is the part of our soul that still reacts with fresh hope and optimism the way a child (who hasn't experienced all of the hurt) explores the world. Getting back to this part of ourselves is much like getting back to our "true" selves, the core, the unique part of us that is undamaged by negative experiences.

- *"I see you, I love you, you are safe."*

- *"I am here for you to love and protect you."*

- *"I will keep us safe and secure."*

- *"You are free to be completely yourself."*

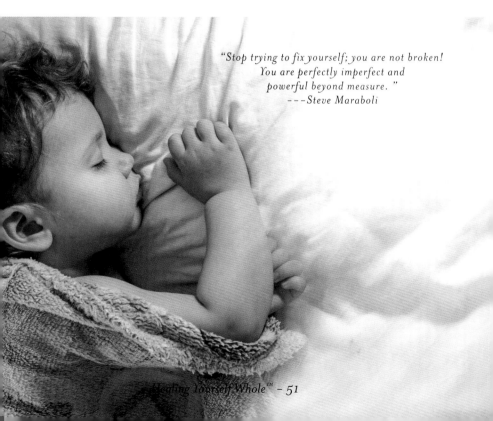

"Stop trying to fix yourself; you are not broken! You are perfectly imperfect and powerful beyond measure. "
---Steve Maraboli

FEELINGS KIT BLEND: PRESENT TIME

"Realize deeply that the present moment is all you have.
Make the now the primary focus of your life."
- Eckhart Tolle

Almond Oil
Neroli
Spruce
Ylang Ylang

I didn't come to "Present Time" until after I had explored many of the singles. Sometime later I re-encountered it, and now I commit to using it when I think it is helpful.

When I first experienced it, it wasn't one that I was most drawn to, but now I have actually started to love that same oil. I don't think of the self-discovery process with oils necessarily as a science, per se. Rather I see it as a skill or art. I think that as I change, my needs for different oils change. And, also sometimes, a particular aroma may not have attracted me at first, but at a later date, that same oil now feels very helpful—and my attraction to it becomes stronger.

It's like eating food. Sometimes my body needs the nourishment of a different vegetable, even though I've had an aversion to it in the past. The power of aromas may not be entirely intuitive at first, so don't be afraid to experiment.

The important thing is to try. Explore what an oil may do and try it for yourself. Always, of course, trust your own judgment. At the same time, be brave enough to take a good look at the emotions that drive your judgment and be willing to re-consider.

In the case of Present Time, I personally wish Gary had named it Now! Eckhart Tolle talks a great deal about the power of now. All we ever have, is now. When we are thinking about memories or worrying about the future, we are no longer aware of now. This one moment keeps moving and changing with our thoughts, perceptions, and emotions. Yet, it is always the same. It is always now.

When applied, Present Time can help you remember that—being aware, awake, and conscious of this moment right here. No matter what you are doing or what's happening around you, this can give you great peace.

Isn't your life worth being present for? Only you can give this gift to yourself. Present Time essential oil can be a powerful reminder to help put things in perspective. It can be a helpful and beautiful reminder to "be here now."

Present Time Placements

Place three drops of Present Time in the palm of your hand and then apply to your thymus (the gland just under your sternum or breastbone).

Present Time Affirmations

To be present is to be in your body, in the now, focused on what is most important to you. When we drift into our past emotional hurts, we lose sight of the now. Use these affirmations to return to the present, relax your thoughts and body, and allowing yourself to return to this now:

- *"I am present here now, I am completely whole, all is well."*

- *"I am willing to be aware and awake right in this moment."*

- *"It is safe to sit and just be."*

- *"As I breathe in this conscious breath, I allow myself to be present in this moment."*

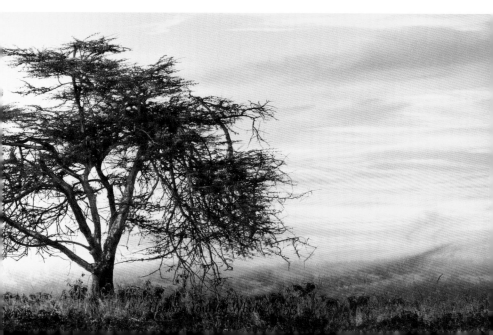

FEELINGS KIT BLEND: RELEASE

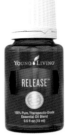

*"Sometimes you don't realize the weight of something
you've been carrying until you feel the weight of its release."*
— Anonymous

I use Release almost every morning. I use it over my liver
and place it there before I start my yoga. I personally like the
idea of moving and sweating toxins out, but with the added
benefit of this oil assisting me in purging my own past
personal traumas. Using them together makes me feel as if
I am doing a great cleanse to my physical, emotional, and
spiritual systems.

*Ylang Ylang
Lavandin
Geranium
Sandalwood
Blue Tansy*

Release Placements

When going through strong feelings of anger, sadness, depression, and
grief, I recommend placing on the liver, soles of the feet, inner elbows,
temples, and above the eyebrows (avoid getting in the eyes).

Release Affirmations

A release is when you allow yourself to escape from the confines of your
past emotional hurts. As you release, you allow yourself to move forward.
You make room for more joy in your life. Repeat these affirmations to gain
release:

- *"I am now free from my old habitual thinking."*

- *"I trust to let go and be fully present in this now."*

- *"I am safe to release whatever no longer serves me."*

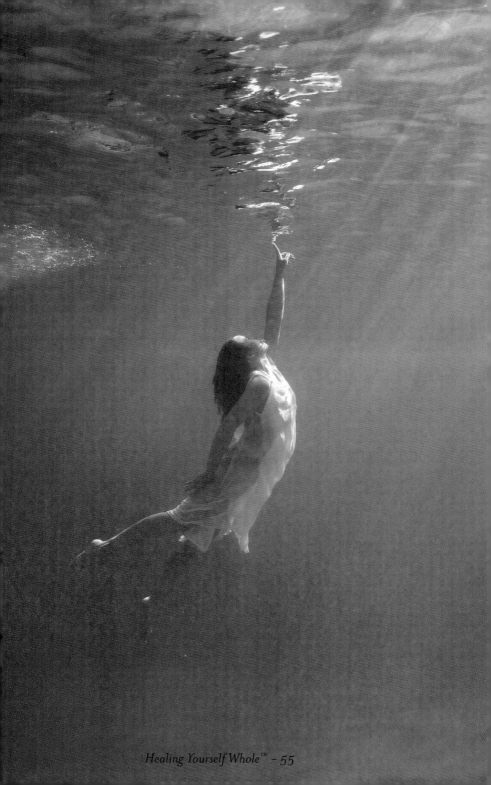

FEELINGS KIT BLEND: VALOR II

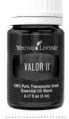

*"Deep down in the human spirit there is a reservoir of courage.
It is always available, always waiting to be discovered."*
- Pema Chodron

Valor is the primary oil I use when having a challenging time, whether I'm stuck in traffic or I'm experiencing something more serious like anxiety attacks. There's a reason it is one of the most popular oils and sells out so quickly. It's potent. It does exactly what the name implies.

*Spruce
Rosewood
Blue Tansy
Frankincense*

Now Valor has been replaced in the Feelings Kit with Valor II. Gary Young formulated this oil with a slightly different profile to bring as many of the benefits as possible without the same tendency for shortage. Everything I describe in affirmations and application can apply to both oil blends.

Valor Placements

I find it best used on the soles of my feet, the palms of my hands, inner wrists, and belly button (navel) and on my solar plexus.

It subtly but profoundly wakes one up out of sluggishness. It gives me courage to go forward (especially when I am afraid, feeling timid or depressed.)

This oil, without a doubt has been my favorite. Although, that said, it's important to note that the more I use oils, the more I change from day to day. My favorite oils change with me as do their benefits and effects.

Life can be challenging—beautiful, exciting, joy-filled, and of course, at times, difficult. Valor can help. Even bringing the bottle up to your nose for 1-2 minutes can affect my mood. It uplifts me and expands my limited thinking to a more grounded and positive mindframe.

To me, it feels like a great friend who reminds me that although I'm made of blood and bone, I'm also made of stardust. And, like everyone, I am connected to everything in the universe. I belong here.

Dictionary definition of valor is strength of mind or spirit that enables a person to encounter danger with firmness; personal bravery.

- "I am made of the same stuff as the universe."

- "I am meant to be here."

- "I am willing to open up to the universe and be guided in my next action."

- "I am open and willing to be guided by the Universal Energy (or with the All That Is, or God)."

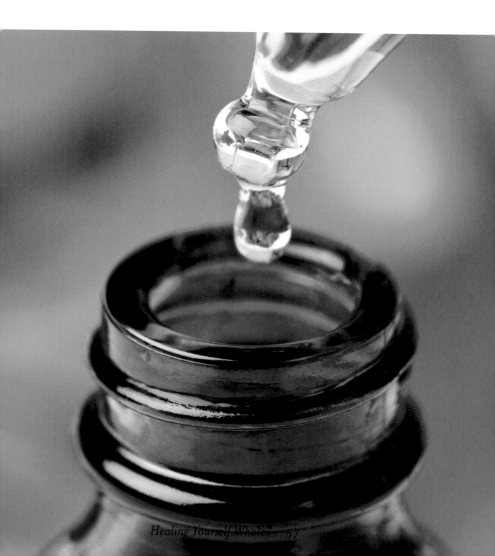

TOOLS FOR YOUR TOOLBOX

Suggestion: write these out and place them where you can see them every day, eg on your fridge, bathroom, dashboard of car.

- Awareness: being fully aware of your emotions.

- Acceptance: allowing them to just be (no stuffing or actioning them away).

- Action: with presence, seeing what you need, applying oils, finding out how to nourish and support more balance in your being and in your life.

Creating a sacred space just for you

Find a space in your home, office, or even outdoors, a space that you can come back to over and over again. A space used only for yourself for honoring your sense of peace, calm, comfort and focus. Make sure it is a place that has enough room for you to sit on the floor, do simple stretches (yoga), relax, nap and even meditate. This is your place to come back home to yourself. A place to use your oils, do your inner work and to allow yourself the freedom of feeling and being.

Suggested things to use to create your sacred space:

- all oils
- diffuser
- live beautiful plants
- cut flowers
- candles
- crystals
- pictures of anyone or anything that brings you great inspiration
- pictures of loved ones, human and/or animal
- any music that brings in more expansive serenity

Get creative, decorate and use anything that you connect with and that brings you joy and peace.

Diet

Emotional upsets and traumas can unbalance the whole system, physically and mentally. It is important to take care of your WHOLE system. This includes healthy eating, fresh vegetables and fruits, plenty of pure water and herbal teas.

Helpful suggestions:

- hot water with lemon first thing in the morning to flush out your system
- please drink at least 8 cups a day of pure water
- eliminate or greatly reduce all sugar, white flours, processed foods and fried foods from your diet
- if you are a meat eater eliminate or greatly reduce all beef, pork and lamb foods from your diet (meats are very acid forming and hard on your digestion)
- if you are vegetarian see if it is possible to eliminate or greatly reduce eggs and dairy from your diet
- consider buying organic green powders ie wheatgrass, barleygrass, spirulina and/or chlorella; drink plain with water or add to fruit or vegetable smoothies
- have the bulk of most of your meals be lightly cooked or raw vegetables and add fresh live sprouts wherever you can

(this is just a suggested outline, please use as a possible guide)

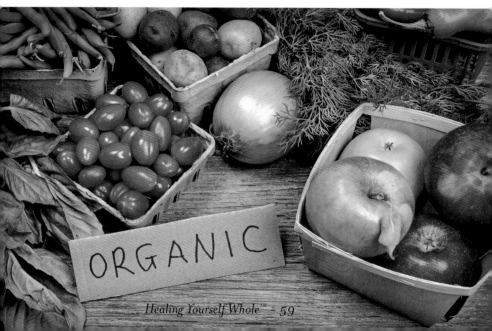

Exercise – moving that body

It is important to move your body, your blood, your muscles and draw fresh air into your lungs each and every day. Exercise can greatly affect our moods and also sleep.

Suggested ways of moving that gorgeous body:

- walk every day for 15-30 minutes around the block or, better still, anywhere in nature eg parks, around lakes, beaches.

- dance, any form or even just turning on the music in your living room and allowing your body to move any way that feels good

- swim

- rollerskate, iceskate, ski (any form)

- join gym or yoga studio

- think outside the box...anything you do that moves your body counts including gardening and cleaning the house

Please use your discretion, bearing in mind your age and ability to move.

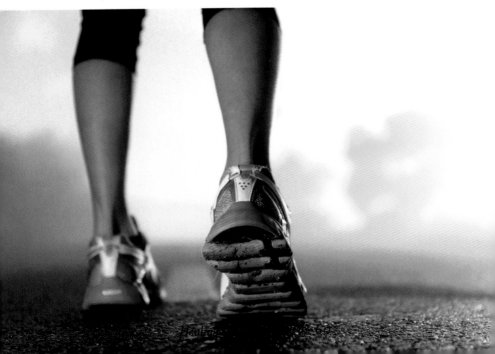

Downtime

It is so important to take time out. We are human beings, not human doings.

Here are some suggestions for downtime but please be creative and find the things that work best for you:

- meditation, praying, chanting etc

- hot baths

- naps (even better if you're lying outside on the earth)

- diary writing

- time with your pet if you have one

- listening to soothing music

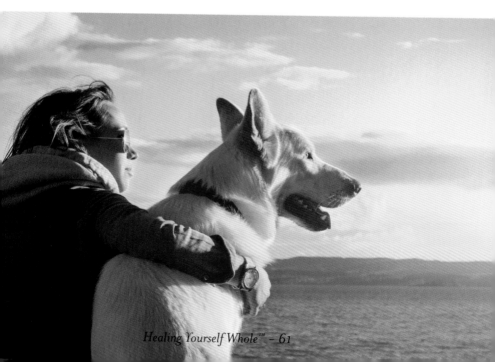

It is important to have fun in your life. Some people think that scheduling fun is a little strange. If you're one of the people who says "fun...what's that?" then chances are you need to schedule some. This means to do something that brings you joy.

Here are some random suggestions:

- visiting museums, art exhibitions

- planning small dinner parties with friends

- cuddling and sharing with the ones you love

- finding inspirational people, reading their biographies or watching movies of their lives

- taking pictures of the world around you

- painting, drawing, ceramics etc.

Explore some place you've never been to in your town and go with a friend. Or you can even make a date with yourself. Planning exciting things for our future makes life a treat and an adventure. Take some time to explore a Farmers Market and buy yourself a new strange fruit or some beautiful fresh flowers. Go to a play, attend a concert or have a nice talk with a friend over lunch. You can do anything that piques your interest. The important thing is simply to incorporate it into your daily life.

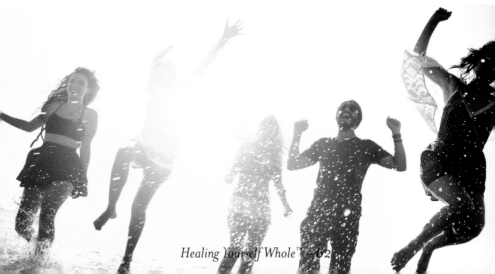

Things to let go of

Be willing to not only go through the physical things you own in your home, but also negative emotional things you may be addicted to. These things clutter and clog up your life.

Suggestions of things to let go of:

- old broken appliances

- clothes that you never wear (offer to charity shops)

- be willing to clean up, refresh or even repaint stale rooms in your home

- give yourself permission to let go of relationships that are habitually harmful to you (without making the other person feel wrong or bad)

- the things you read and the things you watch on TV or the movies... tabloid magazines and gossip TV shows create a difficult dilemma, and even beauty magazines. They might seem attractive, they often fill us with judgmental or even gleeful negative emotions. But, they don't edify or inspire us to forgive, love, or be gentle. They do the opposite. This can have a cumulative negative effect on our well being and outlook. The same is true for violent or horror films. While the scare may feel entertaining- the rush of adrenaline might thrill us - they often play on our negative emotions. Consider where you get your entertainment. Are your attentions feeding your fears and negative emotions? Are they making you more sick or more peace-filled and creative? At the very least, for every negative influence we identify in our lives, it's a good idea to have a positive influence to counter-balance the effects. Think about putting aside the negative influences a little more and drawing upon the positive.

- too much negative news

- indulging in gossiping about other people, tearing them down so that you and who you are gossiping with can feel superior

Showing up for the world by offering your services free of charge, being willing to give and have no expectations of receiving back, is in the end one of the most beautiful gifts you can give yourself and the world around you. By doing this, you are creating not only more love in the world but more self-respect and deep abiding love for oneself.

Suggested ideas:

- volunteer your time to whichever organization calls to you eg
  - elderly care homes
  - hospitals
  - animal shelters
  - homeless shelters

- your service can be anything from picking up trash on the street to smiling and giving an encouraging word to someone who has no home

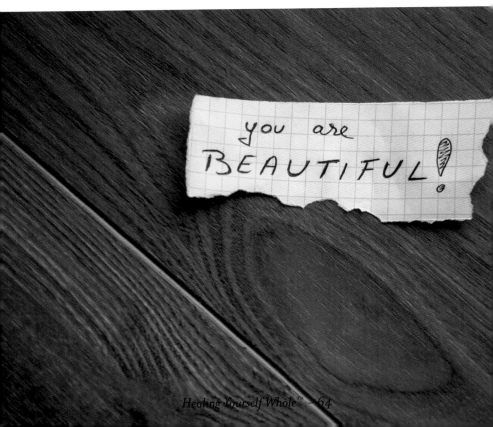

I would like to take this opportunity to thank you for reading and buying this book. I am personally wishing you the very best for your own growth. May you always be open to learning, may you be able to give and receive love from others but especially and most importantly from yourself.